orgasm ...ms

weight... ms

pubertyejaculationsmoking

erectioncircumcisionclitoris

braincellsbulemiacoldsores

shynessconfidentialityacne

erectionmasturbatesteroids

semendevelopmentgspothiv

lovecommunicationanswers

questionserectionssmoking

dietpillsanorexiafriendships

circumcisionpregnantbreast

suicideshynesssteroidscum

orientationdischargenormal

bornagainalcoholhangovers

aphrodisiaclonelinessaddict

I0627212

100 QUESTIONS YOU'D
NEVER
ASK YOUR PARENTS

Elisabeth Henderson

Dr. Nancy Armstrong

&

Uppman Publishing, Richmond

100 QUESTIONS YOU'D NEVER ASK YOUR PARENTS
An Uppman Publishing Book / November 2007

Published by Uppman Publishing
A Division of Colevan International, LLC
Richmond, Virginia

Copyright © 2007 by Elisabeth Henderson

Book Design by Emma DeSilvey

Disclaimer: This book is for informational purposes only and is not intended to constitute medical advice, diagnosis, or treatment. Readers seeking such should direct all personal health questions to a certified physician, licensed counselor or other medical professional.

All rights reserved. No part of this book may be reproduced or transmitted in any form or by any means, electronic or mechanical, including photocopying, recording, or by any information storage and retrieval system, without the written permission of the publisher, except in the case of images which are released for copy, use, modification and printing as specifically and individually specified in the Citations.

ISBN 978-0-615-16518-9

Printed in the United States of America

ERC 4 6 8 10 9 7 5 3

For Cameron & James

In case they never ask

CONTENTS

1. What does an orgasm feel like?   15

2. When I have sex the first time, will people be able to tell?   17

3. Can a gal get pregnant even if she doesn't orgasm?   18

4. What is a wet dream?   20

5. How old do I have to be to buy condoms?   21

6. What is a healthy weight range for me?   22

7. Am I still a virgin if I use a tampon?   27

8. Can a gal get pregnant if she has sex during her period?   29

9. I haven't hit puberty yet...what's wrong with me?   31

10. What's the difference between an orgasm and ejaculation?   33

11. Why does my voice crack?   35

12. Can a guy wear a condom during oral sex?   37

13. Is my penis a normal size?   39

14. Will condoms protect me from all diseases?   40

15. Can I get HIV from kissing? From oral sex?   42

16. How can I get free and confidential STD testing?   44

17. What's the best birth control?   46

18. Does douching after sex prevent pregnancy?   48

19. What are the first signs of puberty?   50

20. Does alcohol really kill brain cells?   52

21. What is pre-ejaculate?   54

22. How can I minimize my acne?   56

23. What is a cold sore?   58

24. Where can I get confidential answers to my questions about sex?   60

25. How much semen is there when a guy cums?   62

26. Is depression and being sad the same?   63

27. What is oral sex?   65

28. Is it normal to get an erection for no reason at all?   66

29. Is smoking safe if I don't inhale?   68

30. How will I know when I'm ready to have sex?   69

31. Are diet pills safe?   72

32. What are anorexia and bulimia?   74

33. Can a virgin get an STD?   77

34. How do I bring up using a condom with my partner?   79

35. Does the first time hurt?   81

36. I'm anorexic...where can I get help?   84

37. How old do I have to be before I can get birth control?   86

38. How can I tell if a guy is a virgin?   88

39. I have no really close friends...what can I do?   89

40. What does a circumcised penis look like? An uncircumcised one?   91

41. With all the condoms out there, how can I know which one to pick?   93

42. How do I put a condom on?   97

43. What is the G-spot?   101

44. What can I do if I just had unprotected sex?   103

45. Do all gals bleed the first time they have sex?   106

46. What do I do now?...I'm pregnant   108

47. What does a vagina look like? A penis?   111

48. How can I lose weight?   114

49. Can a gal get pregnant even if the penis doesn't enter her vagina? 116

50. What is a hickey? 118

51. How do steroids work? 119

52. What does "sexual orientation" mean? 121

53. One of my testicles hangs lower than the other...is this normal? 123

54. What is this discharge? 124

55. How can I get past my shyness? 126

56. Do I have to swallow? 128

57. What is the Morning After Pill? 130

58. How do you kiss? 132

59. What is anal sex? 134

60. I'm unclear about my sexual orientation...what do I do? 136

61. What's the best way to prevent catching an STD? 138

62. What makes a penis get erect? 141

63. What's a clitoris and is it important? 143

64. Do gals ejaculate? 145

65. How often do people have sex? 147

66. If I talk to my doctor about having sex, will she tell my parents? 148

67. Does the withdrawal method work? 150

68. How do I tell my mom that I'm ready to have sex? 151

69. What is a French kiss? 153

70. How can I ask my partner to get tested for STDs? 155

71. Does masturbating have any long-term, negative effects? 157

72. Does the size of a guy's foot really predict his penis size? 159

73. Are my labia normal? 160

74. Does drinking a beer get you less drunk than drinking a shot of liquor? 162

75. What is an aphrodisiac? 164

76. People make fun of me a lot...what can I do? 165

77. What is the difference between HIV and AIDS? 168

78. I've thought about suicide...what should I do? 170

79. How much can I drink before I shouldn't drive? 172

80. Which helps cure a hangover faster – aspirin or coffee? 175

81. What does "popping the cherry" mean? 177

82. How do I do a Breast Self-Exam?   178

83. How can I prevent premature
    ejaculation?   182

84. Can a guy, who hasn't gone through
    puberty, ejaculate?   184

85. What is cunnilingus?   185

86. Are a dildo and a vibrator the same   186
    things?

87. My breasts are lumpy...is this normal?   188

88. She can't get pregnant, so do I need to
    wear a condom when having anal sex?   189

89. Is it ok to go out with my friend's ex if
    she was the one who dumped him?   191

90. Why do my parents always tell me
    to wait before having sex?   193

91. How do I come out to my parents?   196

92. Where can I get free birth control?   198

93. How many times can a gal orgasm
    during sex? A guy?   199

94. I heard pot isn't as dangerous as
    some other drugs...true or false?   201

95. How do I use a female condom?   203

96. Does a guy have to go to a special
    doctor like a gal does?   206

97. I said "no" to sex and my partner
    didn't stop. What do I do now?   207

98. Can a gal get pregnant if a guy
    ejaculates next to her in a pool?   209

99. Can I really die from huffing?   210

100. How long does sex usually last?   213

CITATIONS

EASY GLOSSARY

INDEX

1

What does an orgasm feel like?

Congratulations...you've asked one of the most common questions teens have, so be assured, you're not alone in wondering.

An orgasm is the emotional and physical sensations that are felt at the end of sexual arousal when built-up muscle tension in the body is released. Put simply, it is the climax of the sensations that have been brought about by sexual excitement. Having an orgasm is also sometimes called "cumming".

If you ask ten people what an orgasm feels like, you might get ten different answers because orgasms are very individualistic to each person. For some people, an orgasm involves the whole body – the heart races, the person may vocalize sounds or words, the muscles throughout the body may twitch, breathing can be heavy, and the person may feel flushed. For others, the feeling is more concentrated and remains in the areas of the vagina or penis. While an orgasm will feel different to each person, it is a pleasurable feeling and often associated with euphoria and excitement. It has been described as feeling like a very strong tingling, pleasant and pulsating muscle contractions, or a warm throbbing.

2

When I have sex the first time, will people be able to tell?

No. As much as you may feel like everybody knows, they most likely won't. You won't look any different and there will be no outward physical signs that you've had sex. You may, however, *feel* differently because having sex for the first time is such a big decision. Unless you act differently, however, it is likely that nobody will know.

3

Can a gal get pregnant even if she doesn't orgasm?

Absolutely. That a gal can avoid getting pregnant by not having an orgasm is one of the biggest myths amongst teens. A gal can get pregnant even if she doesn't have an orgasm; an orgasm, or lack of one, has nothing to do with it.

Once a month, a gal ovulates, which means her body releases an egg*. The egg being released is based upon the gal's menstrual cycle, or period, and has nothing to do with whether or not she has an orgasm (a gal does not, in fact, release an egg during orgasm, at all).   If the egg is fertilized with a guy's sperm, the fertilized egg may eventually grow into a baby.   Again, it has nothing to do with whether or not a gal has an orgasm.

*Some gals ovulate more often, some less. Generally speaking, a woman will ovulate once every 28 days.

4

What is a wet dream?

A wet dream is an erotic dream that culminates in orgasm and ejaculation. Wet dreams occur most frequently during a guy's teen and early adult years and are completely involuntary. Some guys wake up as they are ejaculating while others sleep right through it. Wet dreams are commonplace and are no cause for concern; most guys experience them as they go through puberty.

5

How old do I have to be to buy condoms?

There is no age restriction on buying condoms; a person of any age can buy them. Condoms can be purchased at most grocery stores, drugstores and convenience stores and the pharmacist can answer any questions you have about them.

6

What is a healthy weight range for me?

This may seem like a simple question, but it's not! Determining the best weight for your height is based on lots of factors like your body type, amount of fat and muscle, age, gender, etc. Two people of the same height and weight can look and feel dramatically different.

Just imagine two 6'0 guys who both weigh 170 pounds. One is an athlete and all muscle; he's very toned and fit. The other guy has some fat around his stomach and is fairly flabby. Both are the same height and weight, but one is healthy and one is not.

Being in a healthy weight range is important because being too over- or underweight can create health problems. One of the best ways to determine if you are within a healthy weight range is to use a Body Mass Index, or BMI.

BMI indicates how much fat a person has based on his current height and weight. Figures 1-3 can help you determine your Body Mass Index. Using Figure 1, go to the left column and find your height. From your height, scan to the right until you find your weight. Next, scan upward to see you Body Mass Index number.

Now, go to Figure 2 or 3 (depending on if you're a guy or a gal). Find your age along the bottom and your BMI on the left and chart where the two intersect on the graph. Your BMI number will fall within a range of Underweight, Healthy Weight, Overweight or Obese. You can also see what percentile of people you weigh more than (25th percentile means you weigh more than 25% of people who are the same age and gender as you, 75th percentile means you weigh more than 75% of people who are the same age and gender as you, etc.).

Figure 1:
Body Mass Index Values for Use With Ages 2–20 Years

Body Mass Index (kg/m2) — Weight (pounds)

Height (inches)	13	14	15	16	17	18	19	20	21	22	23	24	25	26	27	28	29	30	31	32
48	43	46	49	53	56	59	62	66	69	72	75	79	82	85	88	92	95	99	102	105
49	45	48	51	55	58	61	65	68	72	75	79	82	85	89	92	96	99	103	106	109
50	47	50	54	57	61	64	68	71	75	78	82	85	89	92	96	100	103	107	112	114
51	49	52	56	59	63	67	70	74	78	81	85	89	92	96	100	104	108	112	114	118
52	50	54	58	61	65	69	73	77	81	85	89	92	96	100	104	108	112	116	120	124
53	52	56	60	64	68	72	76	80	84	88	92	96	100	104	108	112	116	120	124	128
54	54	58	62	66	70	75	79	83	87	91	96	100	104	108	112	116	120	124	128	132
55	56	61	65	69	73	77	82	86	90	95	99	103	108	112	116	120	126	130	134	138
56	58	63	67	72	76	80	85	90	94	98	103	107	112	116	120	126	130	134	138	142
57	61	65	70	74	79	83	88	93	97	102	106	112	116	120	126	130	134	138	144	148
58	63	67	72	77	82	86	91	96	101	105	110	116	120	126	130	134	138	144	148	154
59	65	70	75	79	84	89	94	99	104	110	114	120	124	128	134	138	144	148	154	158
60	67	72	77	82	87	92	98	103	108	112	118	124	128	134	138	144	148	154	158	164
61	69	74	80	85	90	96	101	106	112	116	122	128	132	138	144	148	154	158	164	170
62	72	77	82	88	93	99	104	110	114	120	126	132	136	144	148	154	158	164	170	176
63	74	79	85	91	96	102	107	114	118	124	130	136	142	146	152	158	164	170	176	180
64	76	82	88	93	99	105	110	116	122	128	134	140	146	152	158	164	170	176	180	186
65	79	84	90	96	102	108	114	120	126	132	138	144	150	156	162	168	174	180	186	192
66	81	87	93	99	106	112	118	124	130	136	142	150	156	162	168	174	180	186	192	198
67	84	90	96	102	109	116	122	128	134	140	146	154	160	166	172	180	186	192	198	204
68	86	92	99	105	112	120	126	132	138	144	152	158	166	172	178	184	190	198	204	210
69	89	95	102	109	116	122	130	136	142	148	156	162	170	176	184	190	196	204	210	216
70	91	98	105	112	120	126	134	140	146	154	160	168	174	182	188	196	202	210	216	224
71	94	101	108	114	122	130	136	144	150	158	166	172	180	186	194	200	208	216	222	230
72	96	103	110	118	126	134	140	148	154	162	170	178	184	1192	200	206	214	222	228	236
73	99	106	144	122	128	136	144	152	160	166	174	178	190	198	204	212	220	228	236	242
74	102	109	116	124	132	140	148	156	164	172	180	188	194	202	210	218	226	234	242	250

Figure 2: Body Mass Index Chart for GALS

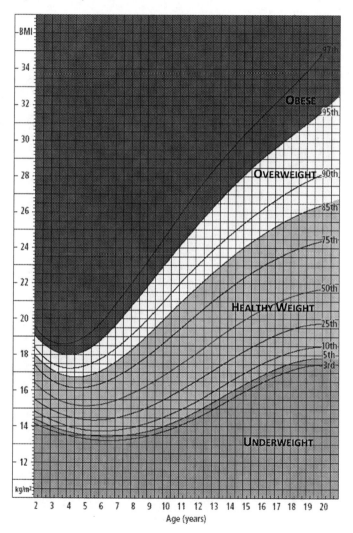

Figure 3: Body Mass Index for GUYS

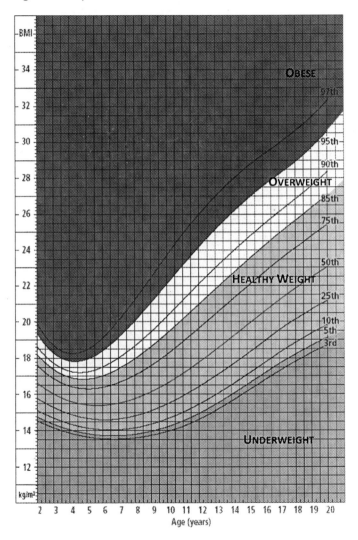

7

Am I still a virgin if I use a tampon?

Yes. A virgin is someone who has never had sexual intercourse. Until you do, you're a virgin; using a tampon doesn't change that.

So then why does this question get asked so often? Virgin gals often have an intact hymen, which is a very thin and flexible membrane, or tissue, that stretches across the opening of the vagina, partially covering it. Some people mistakenly think that a gal loses her virginity if her hymen breaks, and very occasionally, tampon use can break a gal's hymen (just like masturbation, sports, horseback riding or other physical activities could). Using a tampon, even if it were to break the hymen, does not mean a gal isn't a virgin. The only way for a gal to lose her virginity is to have sex.

8

Can a gal get pregnant if she has sex during her period?

While it's rare for a gal to get pregnant during her period, she absolutely could. Usually a gal's period occurs about 14 days after she ovulates. However, if a gal has a short menstrual cycle and long periods, sometimes ovulation (when a gal releases an egg) can overlap with her period. If they do overlap, a gal would be fertile during her period and if she had sex, she could get pregnant.

Also keep in mind that bleeding is not always due to a menstrual period. Sometimes gals bleed small amounts during ovulation as the egg is released and travels down the fallopian tube. This bleeding can be mistaken for a period, but is actually when a gal is most fertile. Remember, unprotected sex at any time is a risk, even during your period. It is always better to use protection and be safe.

9

I haven't hit puberty yet...what's wrong with me?

Puberty isn't a science, and going through it is different for everyone. Some people start early, some start late, some go through it quickly and for others it feels like it takes forever. The good news is that all these differences, while a cause of worry for many teens, are completely normal.

There is no exact age that guys and gals start puberty. Generally speaking, however, gals start puberty between the ages 8 and 13 and guys start a little later, between 9 and 14 (although it can be earlier or later for both groups). For teens that start puberty late, waiting can be difficult, but it is not a reason to worry. "Late bloomers", as they are sometimes called, are almost always healthy.

The age that a person starts puberty is generally dependent on genetics. A gal that develops late may find out that other people in her family also developed later than usual. There are other factors, however, that can cause a small percentage of teens to have delayed development. These factors include malnourishment, chronic illnesses, or problems with the pituitary or thyroid glands. Remember, if you have any concerns at all, talking to a parent or doctor can be a good way to relieve your worries and to make sure that you are developing normally.

10

What's the difference between an orgasm and ejaculation?

Great question. People often use these terms interchangeably, but they are very different acts.

An orgasm is the release of built-up muscle tension in the body that is a result of sexual arousal. Involuntary actions such as quick cycles of pleasurable muscle spasms, vocalizations and euphoria are often associated with having an orgasm. Guys and gals both experience orgasms.

Ejaculation is when semen is ejected from the penis. A guy almost always ejaculates when he has an orgasm. Additionally, a guy could ejaculate without having an orgasm (though this is not common) or orgasm without ejaculating (such as pre-pubescent boys who don't yet produce semen). Most often, however, orgasm and ejaculation occur concurrently in guys.

So what about gals....do they ejaculate? Some people say yes, some say no. Gals definitely have orgasms and all the muscle spasms and pleasurable feelings that are part of them, but whether or not they ejaculate is still undetermined. Many people say they don't and suggest that any wetness that is present during sex is just lubrication that the body makes to accommodate the penis going into the vagina. Others say that gals do ejaculate and that when they do, noticeably more clear fluid comes out of the urethra (fluid that is *not* urine). No explanation has been given for where this fluid comes from, but there remains a controversy nonetheless.

11

Why does my voice crack?

During puberty, guys and gals experience many physical changes. One of the changes a guy goes through is his voice cracking (involuntarily jumping from lower to higher pitches). This is because his larynx, or voice box, is getting bigger and his vocal cords are growing thicker and larger.

Although voice cracking is completely normal, it can be really embarrassing for guys. The good news is, it's just a phase and will pass after a few months. When a guy's voice is done cracking and changing, he will have a deeper, fuller voice.

(Gal's larynxes grow, too, but the change in tone is hardly noticeable, if at all.)

12

Can a guy wear a condom during oral sex?

Absolutely, and it is a good idea for both partners that he do so. STDs such as hepatitis B, genital warts, syphilis, gonorrhea, HIV and herpes can all be spread through oral sex. The best way to reduce the risk of infection is to reduce your exposure, so be smart and be protected. A guy should always wear a condom during oral sex.

When buying condoms for use during oral sex, non-lubricated condoms are the way to go.   The lubrication that comes on some condoms is not something you'd want to taste or ingest!

13

Is my penis a normal size?

Every guy has a different size penis and they are all normal; there is generally no "abnormal' when it comes to penis size. If one guy's eyes are blue and another guy's are brown, both are "normal"; they're just different. It's the same with penises. Even so, penis size is still a big concern for many guys, in part because over the years the size of an average penis has been greatly exaggerated. The true, average length of an erect penis in an adult male is between five and six inches.

14

Will condoms protect me from all diseases?

Condoms are only as good as the people who use them, so they are not foolproof. They can fail due to human error, breakage, and inconsistent or incorrect use. However, when used correctly, condoms are an important and highly effective barrier to the spread of chlamydia, gonorrhea, hepatitis B, HIV and other sexually transmitted diseases (STDs).

As effective as condoms are in preventing STDs that are transmitted by fluid or skin-to-skin contact, not all areas of contact get covered by a condom. If your partner has open sores that are not covered by the condom (from genital warts, syphilis, or herpes, for example) the diseases can still be spread to you. Additionally, condoms made from sheepskin are inadequate in preventing the spread of HIV and other viruses because they have natural pores that the HIV can pass through. If you have sex, latex condoms are your best protection against the spread of disease.

15

Can I get HIV from kissing? From oral sex?

Medical experts agree that under most conditions, you can't become infected with HIV through casual kissing. While saliva does contain HIV, it only contains very small concentrations and not enough to transfer the infection. Therefore casual kissing, such as on the cheek or with a closed mouth, is considered low-risk.

While the exchange of saliva alone poses very little risk, if an infected person's saliva has blood in it, there is a definite risk of transmitting HIV. If both partners have cuts or sores on their lips, mouth or gums (even if they are not readily visible), there is a risk that HIV could be transferred through blood contact. This risk has resulted in the Centers for Disease Control recommending against open-mouth kissing with an infected partner.

Oral sex, either giving or receiving, can result in either partner becoming infected with HIV. So if the person giving oral sex has HIV, it can be transmitted to the receiving person. And if the receiving person has HIV, it can be transmitted to the person performing the oral sex. While using a condom during oral sex reduces the risk of transferring HIV, having oral sex with an infected partner, even with a condom, poses a real and significant risk.

16

How can I get free and confidential STD testing?

Great question. If you think that you've been exposed to a sexually transmitted disease, it is very important that you be tested, not only for your own health, but also for the health of your partner (or future partner). All states offer testing for sexually transmitted diseases through their Department of Health. In some states, testing may be confidential but not free, free but not confidential, or (best case scenario) free and confidential. Minors in many of these states do not need parental consent for examination and treatment. To find a free and confidential clinic in your area, contact your local Department of Health. You may also consider asking your school nurse or your doctor about free clinics, but be sure to ask if your conversation will be kept confidential before you begin. And be proud of yourself; being tested is a responsible and safe choice!

17

What's the best birth control?

"Best" is a relative term, so deciding what the best birth control is depends on (1) what is safest, and (2) what you are personally comfortable with. The only sure way to prevent pregnancy and the spread of most STDs is to not have sex at all (abstinence). All other types of birth control reduce the risks, but they are no guarantee.

There are many types of birth control other than abstinence and each has its own distinct advantages and disadvantages. Remember, however, that birth control is not foolproof and that even people who use it can become pregnant if they use it incorrectly or if something goes wrong (like a condom breaking). Also keep in mind that although all birth control methods can help prevent pregnancy, not all of them help prevent the transmission of STDs.

Birth control pills are one of the most popular forms of contraception because they are easy to take and highly effective. If taken every day as directed, the pill has a 99% success rate in preventing pregnancy. It does not, however, offer any protection against STDs. The condom is also very popular because it is easy to get, inexpensive, and helps protect against the spread of STDs. Typically, condoms have an 85% success rate. Another good alternative is to use *both* the pill and a condom to further reduce the chances of getting an STD or becoming pregnant.

There are many other contraceptives available. You may want to talk to your doctor about what birth control method is best for you.

18

Does douching after sex prevent pregnancy?

No - this is a widespread myth.

Douching is when a gal squeezes a mixture of water, and either a mild soap or vinegar, into her vagina to cleanse it.* It does not prevent pregnancy. In fact, as the solution is sprayed, it may push the sperm further up the vagina, actually increasing the chance of pregnancy. Also, sperm are very fast swimmers, so by the time a gal douches, the sperm could have already reached the cervix. As popular as this myth is among teens, it is completely untrue.

*Douches are pre-mixed, store-bought items and should never be self-made at home.

19

What are the first signs of puberty?

Puberty is the physical transition of a child into an adult that is capable of reproduction. Gals generally start puberty between the ages 8 and 13 and guys generally start later, between the ages of 9 and 14. It is completely normal, however, for some people to start puberty a little earlier or later.

In gals, the first sign of puberty is usually breast development, sometime around the age of 10 or 11. Six to twelve months later, pubic hair begins to grow and fill in. Around the age of 12 or 13, gals can also expect to start menstruating, or having a period.

In guys, the first sign of puberty is usually the testes, or "balls" getting larger. Next comes penis growth, which continues until a guy is about 18 years old. Soon after the penis starts to grow, pubic hair also begins to grow, followed by body and facial hair over the next few years. A guy will also experience his voice "cracking" as his voice deepens to its final, adult tone.

Both guys and gals will grow taller and their body shapes will change as they go through puberty. They may also experience body odor and acne during this time.

Remember, it is very normal for people to begin developing at different ages and to continue at different rates. If you have any concerns however, talking to a parent, counselor or doctor can be a good way to alleviate and address them.

20

Does alcohol really kill brain cells?

Whether or not alcohol actually kills brain cells is a hot topic of research today. For every study that says alcohol does kill brain cells, another one says it does not. The generally accepted consensus, however, is that while alcohol does not kill brain cells*, it does damage the fibers that carry information between the brain cells, thereby impairing communication between the cells. Although there is still some disagreement over this, all studies agree that alcohol definitely has significant and negative effects on the brain, damaging both its structure and its functions.

Some of the damage to the brain is noticeable after one or two drinks and then resolves once the drinking stops. Examples of this short-term damage are blurred vision, slurred speech, weakened memory, slow reaction times, and difficulty walking and driving. Other brain damage occurs from heavy, long-term drinking and persists even after a person is sober. This type of brain damage includes shrinkage of the brain as well as trouble with learning, memory, movement and coordination.

Teens that drink alcohol may interrupt important brain development, possibly leading to mild cognitive impairment and negatively affected academic achievement. So, although the controversy over whether or not alcohol kills brain cells is still being debated, the negative effects it can have in both the short- and long-term are crystal clear.

*Alcohol does kill the brain cells of a developing fetus if a pregnant woman drinks.

21

What is pre-ejaculate?

Pre-ejaculate is the clear, slippery, slightly thick fluid that comes out of a penis when a guy is sexually aroused. It is usually secreted during masturbation, foreplay, or any time before a guy ejaculates, or "cums", and is therefore sometimes called "pre-cum". Some guys produce very small amounts and some guys produce a lot.

Pre-ejaculate serves two purposes. First, it gets the urethra ready for the ejaculation of semen. Second, it lubricates the movement of the penis during sexual arousal.

Pre-ejaculate contains enough sperm to get a gal pregnant and in an infected person, will also contain HIV, so play it safe around pre-ejaculate!

22

How can I minimize my acne?

Acne usually develops during puberty and can be very upsetting to guys and gals who have it. It develops when a person's pores get clogged with oil and dead skin cells, as well as by the hormonal changes that occur during puberty. In teens, acne often appears on the face, neck, upper back, shoulders and chest. Some people have only a few pimples while others have many. Most people's acne fades over time, but there is no way to know how long that will take.

Treatments for acne work by reducing oil production, opening up the pores, and fighting bacteria that causes infections in the pores. To help prevent, control, or minimize acne, follow a good skin care routine. Remove excess oil and dead skin by washing your face (or other affected area) twice a day with soap and water. If oil is still a problem, a gentle astringent can help wipe it away (you can find them wherever cosmetics are sold). Some people also use a mild scrub or exfoliant to open the pores and further remove dead skin cells. Next, make sure any moisturizer you use is oil-free and contains an antibacterial agent to further reduce the outbreaks. Also, minimize your use of cosmetics. Finally, there are some great over-the-counter acne lotions that help dry up excess oil, while others are medicated and prescription-only. If the over-the-counter methods don't control your acne, a dermatologist (skin specialist) can help determine which treatment may be best for you.

And remember...if you do get a pimple, never pick or squeeze it; it will go away faster if you don't!

23

What is a cold sore?

Cold sores, also known as herpes or fever blisters, are caused by the herpes simplex virus. They look like small blisters that appear on the lips, inside the mouth, and adjacent to the mouth. Cold sores usually persist for 10-14 days.

When a cold sore appears, the area will first become tingly and sensitive to touch and a person will be able to feel (but not see) a small hard spot. Usually by day three, tiny blisters have formed. These blisters sometimes fill with fluid before splitting and becoming painful and raw. Eventually, the area will begin to scab over and heal itself.

Cold sores are very common and are contagious if you come into contact with one. A person that has an active cold sore should avoid kissing, sharing a glass or utensils, and touching the cold sore and then touching someone else. He should also wash his hands regularly to prevent the spread of the herpes virus to other parts of his body, or to someone else. And no matter what, a person with a cold sore should never pick at it. Doing so will slow down the healing process and increase the chance of spreading the virus.

Once a person has been infected with the herpes virus, he has it forever; cold sores can't be cured. At random times throughout the person's life, a cold sore may simply recur spontaneously. While this can be aggravating, the good news is that a cold sore's pain, frequency and duration can be lessened with medication. Over-the-counter medications are available at drugstores, or there are also some really great prescription medications available through your doctor.

24

Where can I get confidential answers to my questions about sex?

Confidential counseling about sex and other topics is available to teens through many sources. It would be an oversight to not mention the internet, but the internet has a lot of incorrect information on it, so be careful. Also keep in mind that the pages you visit on the internet are logged in your computer, so it's not confidential; if someone really wanted to know what you were looking at online, they could find out. Besides, with such an important topic, talking to a person would probably be much more beneficial.

Obviously parents, close relatives and friends would all be helpful, but if you want confidentiality, there are other places you could go, as well. Your counselor at school will likely keep your conversation confidential as long as you are not talking about hurting yourself or others. Also, many doctors will treat their teen patients confidentially, while others require a parent's permission before doing so; ask your doctor about her policies. Public health clinics also offer confidential advice about sexual health and other health matters, at reduced rates to teens. If you're not sure whether your conversation with someone will be treated confidentially, ask them upfront, before you discuss details.

25

How much semen is there when a guy cums?

The average amount of semen per ejaculation is one to two teaspoons.

26

Is depression and being sad the same?

Sadness is a natural reaction to painful experiences or situations. It is a healthy way to experience your feelings and adjust to a disappointment, change or loss. Being sad is part of a healing process people go through and the feeling usually lasts anywhere from a few hours to a few days. Everybody gets sad sometimes.

Depression is very different from sadness. It is a state of despair that lasts for more than two weeks and is so severe that it disrupts a person's life. The person's social interactions, daily schedule and activities are impacted because of the extreme unhappiness. People who are depressed may describe "feeling sad for no reason" and can feel unmotivated, irritable, tired and uncaring about things that were once important to them. Depressed people may also have a noticeable change it appetite, problems sleeping, and trouble concentrating. They often describe feeling like there is no hope. Although it is a serious condition that requires treatment, with help, depression can be overcome and a person can live a happy and healthy life.

27

What is oral sex?

Oral sex is when a person's mouth or tongue is used to stimulate another person's genitalia (including a guy's penis, a gal's clitoris and vagina, and the anus). When oral sex is performed on a guy it is called fellatio; when it is performed on a gal it is called cunnilingus. Both are sometimes referred to as "going down" on a partner.

28

Is it normal to get an erection for no reason at all?

Yes, it is completely normal to get an erection for no reason at all. Almost every guy experiences spontaneous erections as he goes through puberty because of all the hormonal changes that are occurring in his body. While it's normal to get spontaneous erections, it doesn't make them any less embarrassing to the person experiencing them.

Since they're spontaneous, there's no telling when a spontaneous erection may occur – in the middle of class, at sports practice, at dinner – there's just no way to predict. The good news is, the more a guy ignores it and thinks of mundane things, the quicker it will end (hopefully). Until it does, a guy can conceal a spontaneous erection with baggy clothes or by holding something in front of his body, like a book. Also, guys tend to get less spontaneous erections after they've recently ejaculated.

29

Is smoking safe if I don't inhale?

No, smoking is never safe. When you smoke, nicotine enters the bloodstream through the lungs. Even if you don't inhale, nicotine can be absorbed through the lining of the mouth. This can eventually lead to cancer of the mouth, esophagus, larynx, lungs, bladder or pancreas. It can also lead to sinus disease, emphysema, chronic bronchitis, coronary heart disease and other diseases. Whether or not you inhale, smoking is harmful to your health and could eventually even result in death.

30

How will I know when I'm ready to have sex?

Great question. Having sex for the first time is a huge decision. Asking yourself if you're ready means you already recognize this and are carefully thinking it through.

Everybody is different and knowing when is right for you is an individual decision. There is no set age or time that defines it. Keep in mind that while you are the only person who will know when you're ready, you may not recognize if you *aren't* ready. There are some people who thought they were ready and later wished they had waited a while longer. Be sure you are comfortable with your decision before you do anything because you can always have sex later, but you can never go back.

When making your decision, you will have to weigh a lot of important considerations. Some questions you could ask yourself to help you decide if you are ready to have sex or not are:

1. Does my decision coincide with my morals, character, and family values?

2. Do I know how to get, and properly use, birth control?

3. Could I have any regrets about my decision later?

4. Am I emotionally ready to share myself in such an intimate and important way?

5. Can I openly discuss my feelings and concerns with my partner?

6. Am I considering having sex because I want to, or because I feel pressured to?

7. Will I be proud of myself and my decision if people find out about it?

8. Am I ready to take responsibility for possible consequences of my decision (disease or pregnancy)?

Talking to a parent, other close family member, counselor or doctor could help you make this very important decision. Although talking about sex might be hard to do, it is easier than regretting the decision you make, no matter which one it is. Get advice from people who love, support and want the best for you. And be sure before you do anything.

31

Are diet pills safe?

Diet pills, or weight-loss pills, can be very appealing to guys and gals who want to lose weight quickly. They seem to be an easy solution, but there is a lot to know about diet pills before you take them. The facts indicate that over-the-counter diet pills are, generally, either: (1) safe, but unlikely to cause weight loss or (2) slightly effective in speeding up weight loss but very harmful to the body.

Diet pills work in one of three ways. They can suppress your appetite, increase your metabolism, or block your absorption of nutrients (such as fat or carbohydrates). Weight-loss pills aren't subject to the same regulations as prescription drugs or other over-the-counter medications, so they can be sold even if their effectiveness is extremely limited. In addition, many diet pills have unsafe side effects such as: constipation, bloating, insomnia, diarrhea, nausea, indigestion, vomiting, heart palpitations and stroke. Even some deaths have been attributed to the use of diet pills.

Sometimes a doctor may prescribe a safe, regulated weight-loss medication to a person who is so extremely overweight that her health is jeopardized. These medications are different than over-the-counter pills and under the supervision of a doctor, can be safe and effective. However, for the average person who just wants to lose some weight, the best thing to do is make lifestyle changes. Eat healthier, lower-calorie foods, minimize your portion sizes and exercise regularly. Remember, there is no magic pill; over-the-counter diet pills are generally not effective and can cause more harm than good.

32

What are anorexia and bulimia?

Anorexia and bulimia are both eating disorders. People who have anorexia or bulimia have a distorted body image, meaning they don't see their body as it really is. They generally see themselves as overweight or unattractive, no matter how skinny or attractive they really are. Anorexia and bulimia are also characterized by an obsessive fear of weight gain. They are both psychological conditions wherein people use food to address their emotional pain, but they are characterized by physical symptoms.

People who are anorexic eat very little and essentially starve themselves. They may also exercise excessively in order to keep weight off or use diet pills or laxatives for the same reason. Anorexics maintain a body weight that is at least 15% less than their healthy body weight range. In addition to losing too much weight to be healthy, anorexia is also very harmful in other ways. Anorexics may experience heart failure, stunted growth, thinning hair, problems with their immune system, changes in brain structure and even death.

People who are bulimic eat a large amount of food and then purposefully vomit it up. This pattern of excessive, uncontrolled overeating followed by purging is called binge eating. Bulimics may also purge their body of the food by using laxatives, medications, or by exercising excessively. Bulimics sometimes use binge eating as a response to stress, depression or self-esteem issues. Unlike anorexics, bulimics are often within a normal weight range and appear to be physically healthy. They often, however, experience an irregular heartbeat, heartburn, constipation, weakness, exhaustion, and heart attacks.

They also often have cavities, erosion of tooth enamel, a sore throat, abdominal pain, ulcers, rupturing of the stomach and increased risk of suicidal behaviors. Like anorexia, bulimia is a serious and life-threatening disorder.

Approximately ten percent of people with anorexia and bulimia die directly from the diseases or from their harmful effects. The good news is that support is available and both anorexia and bulimia are treatable with the right help.

33

Can a virgin get an STD?

Yes, a virgin can get an STD. Sexually transmitted diseases, or STDs, can be transferred through sexual intercourse, as the name suggests, or through sexual touching. Anytime you have skin-to-skin contact with an infected partner, you are at risk for getting an STD. Diseases such as HPV (also known as Human Papilloma Virus or genital warts), chlamydia and genital herpes, among other diseases, can all be spread without having sex. So, for example, if a guy has warts on his hand and masturbates his partner, he can spread the infection. Or if a gal has a cold sore and performs oral sex on her partner, she can spread the herpes infection to her partner's genital area. Keep in mind that a person with an STD may not know he has it because STDs can lie latent in the body for up to a year before showing any symptoms.

Some STDs can also be passed from a mother to her fetus either in the uterus or during childbirth. This is another way a virgin could have an STD.

34

How do I bring up using a condom with my partner?

Talking about how to have safer sex with your partner is very important. While it might be slightly embarrassing at first, it is absolutely necessary if you're going to share in the intimacy and responsibility of sex. One of the easiest ways to bring it up is to just do it – jump in with two feet. Highlight the importance of protecting yourselves against diseases which one of you may already have (even if you haven't seen any symptoms of it, yet). Also discuss the importance of protecting against an unplanned pregnancy. Talk about the responsibilities that would arise if you didn't use a condom and you either spread an infection to your partner or got pregnant. Using a condom will protect both you and your partner, and who doesn't want that? Bringing up the topic of using a condom may be a little awkward at first, but you and your partner will both be glad you did!

35

Does the first time hurt?

For a guy, the first time he has sex should not hurt. It may be a nervous time, but it should not be a painful time. If it is painful, something may be wrong and he should see his doctor for an exam.

For a gal, the first time may be anywhere from pleasurable to painful. What the experience is like depends on a lot of factors including the gal's body and the amount of foreplay involved.

If a gal does experience pain during sex, there could be a few reasons for it. First, if there is pain as the penis initially enters the vagina, the problem is probably due to not having enough lubrication. These are sensitive areas and friction can hurt, which is why the body naturally gets wet and slippery through sexual arousal. Spending a little more time with foreplay to help the vagina become lubricated naturally, or using an artificial lubricant such as KY Jelly, will help correct the problem. Another possible reason for pain would be if the gal's hymen is still intact. If it is, it may be painful as the hymen stretches and breaks (there will also be some bleeding). To help ease any discomfort, your partner should go slowly and in small increments as opposed to pushing fast all at once. A third possible reason for pain would be if something is wrong, like if the gal has a yeast infection or an STD. Any pain experienced during sex because of an infection will last until the infection is treated.

You don't have to feel pain during sex; it is supposed to be enjoyable. If pain occurs at all, it should only be slight and temporary. It is important to talk with your partner and ensure that you are both physically and emotionally comfortable before continuing. And remember, you only have one "first time". Make sure you have thought your decision through and if you decide you're ready to have sex, protect yourself and your partner with a condom.

36

I'm anorexic...where can I get help?

Talk to someone you trust. Anorexia can be overcome, but you'll need some help to do it. Your best choice is to talk to an adult because they'll have, or can get, the resources and support you'll need to get well. Your parents, doctor, school counselor or a trusted family friend are just a few people you may consider going to. They will want to help you and will be glad you confided in them.

If you're not ready to talk to someone yet, an excellent resource is the ANAD – National

Association of Anorexia Nervosa and Associated Disorders (www.anad.org). You'll find links for treatment and referrals as well as contact information for support groups, which are organized by state. There is also a message board and chat rooms for more information and support. Additionally, almost every city has treatment programs at eating disorder treatment centers. If you need more help in finding one, ANAD can help with that, also. And a big "pat-on-the-back" for seeking help because with it, you *can* get well again.

37

How old do I have to be to get birth control?

Birth control comes in many forms: condoms, the pill, abstinence, diaphragms, IUDs and the ring, to name a few. You're never too young to practice abstinence and you can get a condom at any age. As for prescription birth control methods such as the pill, ring, diaphragm, etc., the age you can get them depends on which state you live in. In many states, you don't have to be very old. In fact, a lot of doctors prescribe the pill to teen gals in order to reduce the pain and menstrual flow of their periods. Your doctor can help determine what birth control is most appropriate for you given your age and circumstances. And don't be afraid to ask – in most states, a conversation about birth control is confidential and your doctor will not tell anyone you asked (to be sure, though, ask your doctor what her policy is).

38

How can I tell if a guy is a virgin?

The only way to find out if a guy is a virgin is to ask him. There is no other way – physically, appearance, or otherwise – to tell if a guy is a virgin.

39

I have no really close friends...what can I do?

First, know that you are in the company of thousands of guys and gals who feel exactly the same way. While it may seem like everybody else is overflowing with close and meaningful friendships, you are not alone; many people feel the exact same way as you.

So, how can you make new friends? First, remember that the more people you're around, the more opportunities you have to meet people. Get out, even if you have to go alone, and put yourself around other people: a baseball game, an after-school club, the local, fun place to hang-out, the park, the zoo, a lake, the pool...just go! Get out there! Next, be friendly. There is not a person in the world that has too many friends, so say "hello" to someone. Find a common interest (the game's score, an activity, the menu, the lifeguard's haircut) and begin a conversation. It goes without saying that you should be careful about whom you approach, but every new friendship begins with a first "hello". The more of these you have, the more friends you'll make. And remember to just be yourself, because you're great the way you are. Now all you have to do is show people who that great person is!

40

What does a circumcised penis look like? An uncircumcised one?

The difference between a circumcised and an uncircumcised penis has to do with foreskin. Foreskin is a loose fold of skin that covers the tip of the penis; every baby boy is born with it. Some parents have the foreskin of their baby removed by a doctor when the baby is only a few days old. This act of cutting off the foreskin and removing it is called circumcision.

So, a circumcised penis has no extra skin covering the tip of the penis. The tip (otherwise known as the glans or head) is fully visible in both the flaccid (limp) and erect positions. An uncircumcised penis has its foreskin intact. When the penis is limp, the foreskin covers the tip of the penis, much like a turtle in its shell. When the penis is erect, the foreskin naturally gets pulled back off the tip of the penis as it enlarges.

Both circumcised and uncircumcised penises are "normal" and "ok"; one is not more "normal" than the other.

41

With all the condoms out there, how can I know which one to pick?

Great question. Condoms are the only protection that reduces the spread of STDs *and* helps prevent pregnancy, so using them is a very responsible act. There are male and female condoms available, but let's talk about male condoms. For more about female condoms, see question #95.

It used to be that a condom was just a condom, but not anymore. Now, there are many different options for condoms users, and many things to consider:

1. *Material:* Condoms are made from one of three materials: latex, polyurethane, or lambskin. All three are equally effective in protecting against pregnancy, but they protect differently against STDs.

> a. Latex – What most people think of when they think "condom"; made of rubber; good protection against STDs, easy to find and most widely used; about $9 per dozen; can only be used with water-based lubricants; bad taste for use with oral sex

> b. Polyurethane – Newest on the market; made from plastic; good protection against STDs, are slightly less flexible than latex and may require more lubrication; are thinner than latex and therefore increase sensitivity for some users; about $14 per dozen; can be used with oil or water-based lubricants; no bad taste

> c. Sheepskin – Oldest on the market; made of lamb intestine (not sheepskin); does not protect against STDs; contain natural, small pores that *allow* the

transmission of viruses that cause STDs; the thinnest condom so it generally feels the most natural; about $20 per dozen; can be used with oil or water-based lubricants

2. *Size:* Condoms come in a standard size, a smaller size which is a little more snug, and a mega or magnum size which is about 2mm wider than the standard size.

3. *Lubrication:* Lubrication refers to a substance that makes the condom easier to put on and for some people, more comfortable to use. Pre-lubricated condoms come with lubricant already inside the condom. If you get condoms that are not pre-lubricated, you can always add a lubricant when you put the condom on. Water-based lubricants work well with all condoms; oil-based ones break down some condoms.

4. *Ribbed:* Condoms that are textured with ribs or bumps to increase sensation.

5. *Shape:* Straight Sides, Form Fitted (indented below the head of the penis), or Flared (wider over the head of the penis), amongst others

6. *Color & Flavor:* Most condoms are clear with no flavor, but you can buy colored or flavored ones for fun.

7. *Brand:* Stick with a name brand.

Remember, if you get to the pharmacy and don't know which to buy, or can't make sense of all the options, the pharmacist can discreetly help you decide which condom is right for you.

42

How do I put a condom on?

Everyone is nervous the first time they put a condom on in front of, or for, their partner. If, however, you're comfortable having sex with your partner, hopefully you are comfortable enough to put a condom on in front of her! And if you mess up, it's no big deal; just throw the condom out, get another one, and try again.

A little practice before you start can help a lot. A guy can practice putting a condom on himself; gals can practice on a banana.

(Really, it is good practice!)

So here's what you need to know:

1. The penis must be erect.

2. Check the expiration date on the packet.

3. Open the condom packet, being sure not to tear the condom.

4. If you want to add lubrication to the inside of the condom to increase sensitivity and reduce friction, put in a drop or two.

5. Most condoms have a reservoir tip to hold the ejaculation and you don't want air to be in there when you put the condom on (air trapped in a condom could cause it to break). So, squeeze the tip on the condom between your thumb and forefinger and place it over the head of the erect penis. If the condom does not have a reservoir tip, make sure to leave about half an inch of space at the tip of the penis to collect the semen. Also make sure the roll is on the outside (that the condom is not inside-out, or you won't be able to easily roll it down the penis).

6. Still squeezing the tip of the condom, use your other hand to unroll the condom down the length of the penis. Make sure to unroll it all the way and to cover as much as the penis as possible. Smooth out any air bubbles by rubbing your hand down the penis a few times.

7. If you want to, you can add more lubricant on the outside of the condom to ease the friction that will be against the penis as it slides in the vagina.

8. If the condom comes off or breaks during sex, withdraw the penis and condom immediately, wash the penis to remove any remaining sperm, and put on a new condom.

After ejaculation, while the penis is still partially erect, withdraw the penis from the vagina. Be sure to hold the condom in place at the base of the penis as you withdraw or you could pull out of the condom, accidently leaving it in the vagina. Remove the condom only after you've fully withdrawn and keep it and the penis away from your partner's body so no sperm transfer to her. Wrap the condom in tissue and throw it in a trashcan (it'll clog a toilet).

Remember - never, ever use a condom more than once, never store a condom in your wallet or glove box (the heat is very bad for them) and look for the expiration date before using a condom.

43

What is the G-spot?

The G-spot (short for Gräfenberg spot) is a highly sensitive area in the vagina that is especially responsive to sexual stimulation. It is a one to three centimeter-long area along the upper vaginal wall (the side closest to the belly) that begins an inch or two from the opening. It will feel bumpy or like it has ridges. When a gal is aroused, the G-spot is said to swell slightly.

There is a lot of controversy about whether the G-spot actually exists. Doctors and scientists generally agree that such a uniquely sensitive area does not exist, but the general consensus of the public is that it does.

44

What can I do if I just had unprotected sex?

First, you're smart to recognize that you need to take action to protect yourself as much as you can, even after the fact. By having unprotected sex, you've exposed yourself to many risks, with sexually transmitted diseases and pregnancy being the biggest two. The best you can do now is to take precautions that will protect you and your partner in the future.

Next, know that washing, rinsing or douching will not help prevent pregnancy and will not wash away any STDs. Since you may now be pregnant, you'll need to consider emergency contraception. Emergency contraception, otherwise known as the Morning After Pill, can help you avoid pregnancy if it is taken within 72 hours of having unprotected sex. It works best within 24 hours, however, and is about 90% effective. You can get the Morning After Pill from your doctor or at most pharmacies. If you decide against taking this pill, make sure to take a pregnancy test in a few weeks to determine if you are pregnant.

Next, you'll need to find out if you or your partner has transmitted an STD to one another. If you are having sex with someone, you have probably already discussed your health and theirs, but if you didn't, you *really* need to now. Talk about if either of you currently has an STD and if one of you does, you'll both need to get medical treatment immediately. Keep in mind that some infected people do not know that they have an STD and, therefore, they unknowingly transmit it to their partner. Also keep in mind that many STDs do not show their symptoms right away and some are not detectable without the aid of a doctor. For these reasons, you'll need to examine yourself regularly for symptoms of STDs for the next few months and have a doctor examine you to determine if you are infected. Make sure to take this essential step in protecting yourself and your partner for the future. Also, make very sure to use protection going forward (especially during the time before you see the doctor) so you don't further risk spreading STDs.

Having unprotected sex is a risky thing to do. Putting a condom on may take an extra minute and may not seem like as much fun as having sex without one, but if you do have unprotected sex, you're exposing yourself to pregnancy, STDs and months of worry, tests and concern until a doctor can determine if you are healthy or not. It only takes one instance of unprotected sex to give you an STD that will last a lifetime. In the future, protect yourself and your partner by using a condom.

45

Do all gals bleed the first time they have sex?

Some gals bleed the first time they have sex and some gals don't. Just like with every other aspect of sex, the answer depends on the person. Whether or not a gal bleeds has nothing to do with her virginity (or lack of virginity). You cannot tell if a gal is a virgin by whether or not she bleeds; some virgins will and some virgins won't.

Bleeding after having sex for the first time occurs when the hymen is stretched, or broken. If a gal's hymen had previously been broken (by rough exercise, tampon use or something else) she will not experience bleeding after having sex for the first time. However, if her hymen was intact prior to having sex, she will have some bleeding. A gal can expect anywhere from a few drops to a light flow of blood when her hymen is broken.

46

What do I do now?...I'm pregnant

Gals who find out they're pregnant run the gamut of emotions from excited and thankful to terrified and surprised. Depending on your situation, you may experience some or all of these emotions. No matter the circumstances, every gal who finds out she's pregnant faces similar new responsibilities.

First, get support. This is one of the most life-changing experiences you will ever face. You will need the support of someone who loves you as you make decisions that will affect your future. If you were buying a car, picking a college to attend, or getting a job, you'd seek support and advice from knowledgeable people. Pregnancy is far more significant than any of those decisions, so make sure you talk with someone you respect, love, and trust.

Next, get educated. Talk with your parents, partner, doctor, school nurse, and/or counselor. You will be making choices that you'll live with for the rest of your life, so be sure to know how they may affect you. Think about the emotional, physical, social, medical, financial, educational, and life-style changes that will come with the decisions you make.

Remember, no choice may feel totally right, but talking it through and earnestly weighing the options will help you determine what is best under the circumstances. The choices are complicated and deeply personal. And your decisions will have a life-changing impact on you and the baby, not just now, but for years to come. Think about the consequences of your choices and what is best in the long term. Get support, get educated and make the best decision possible for both you and the baby. And no matter what choice you make, you will need medical care immediately.

Finally, if getting pregnant was not something you planned, use protection in the future to avoid being in the same situation.

47

What does a vagina look like? A penis?

A guy's genitals are pretty straight forward. First, there is a penis. The penis is made up of two parts: the shaft and the glans. The shaft is the main part of the penis and the glans is the tip (or head of the penis). Next, there are two testicles (sometimes called balls) that are contained within a scrotum (the sack that holds the testicles). There is also the perineum, which is the area of skin between the scrotum and anus. Finally, there is the anus.

A gal's genitals require a little more explanation. The exterior genitalia, called a vulva, is comprised of many parts. There are "outer lips" (labia majora) that protect all the other parts of the vulva. Within these lips are another set of lips called the "inner lips", or labia minora. The inner lips are softer and engorge with blood when a gal is aroused. Within the inner lips, at the very top where they come together, is a clitoral hood. The clitoral hood covers and protects the clitoris. The clitoris is a sexual organ that has about twice as many nerve endings as the head of a penis and therefore is very sensitive to, and becomes stimulated by, sexual touch. The clitoris is approximately the size of a pencil eraser, but can be smaller or larger from gal to gal. Below the clitoris is the urinary opening and below the urinary opening is the vaginal opening (or vagina). The area of skin between the vagina and the anus is called the perineum. Finally, there is the anus.

Genitals of both guys and gals can look dramatically different from one person to another. It is very normal for penises to vary in length, width, color and shape. It is also normal for scrotum to look different from one guy to the next. In gals, it is common for there to be wide variations in the appearance of the vulva; differences in length, shape, fullness, texture, color and elasticity are all quite common.

48

How can I lose weight?

With all the infomercials, pills, gadgets, diets and hype in the media, the world of weight loss has become a circus. Unfortunately, most of these "quick fixes" will leave you out of a lot of money and time and with a roller-coaster weight that goes up and down. Fad diets can actually make it harder for you to lose weight because your body will not want to "yo-yo" with up and down weight loss anymore and will therefore fight against any weight loss at all. Managing your weight is about permanently changing your unhealthy eating habits and adopting lifelong, healthy habits that you can maintain.

The good news is that you can lose weight without spending a lot of money and wasting a lot of time. The answer is very straight forward: take in fewer calories than you put out. In other words, eat less and exercise more. It sounds overly simple, but in the end, this is the healthiest and most consistent way to lose weight and keep it off.

Lessen your portions, choose healthier foods, and choose exercise routines that burn calories. Some exercises or levels of exercise build muscle instead of burning calories, so talk to your doctor about which exercises are best for you. Your doctor can also help you determine what a healthy weight for you is, what portion sizes are best for you, how much you can realistically expect to lose and in what amount of time. Slow and steady wins the race in this case – good luck!

49

Can a gal get pregnant even if the penis doesn't enter her vagina?

Yes. Sperm are very good swimmers and it is their "job" to swim around until they find an egg to penetrate. Even if the penis doesn't enter the vagina, if the pre-ejaculate or ejaculate (cum) gets anywhere near the vagina, the sperm can find their way in and up to an awaiting egg. Inserting fingers that previously touched semen into the vagina, or ejaculating just outside of the vagina, are examples of how a gal could get pregnant without a penis entering the vagina. Anytime there is sperm present, it is important that both partners take care to not transfer it into the vagina, or anywhere near it.

50

What is a hickey?

A hickey is a temporary bruise that is left on the skin. It is caused when forceful sucking or biting, while kissing, breaks blood vessels beneath the skin. Hickeys are red and purple in color (like any other bruise) and last for about 3-5 days, depending on their size and severity. There is no way to make hickeys disappear faster, but wearing makeup or covering them with a collared shirt can help conceal them from view.

51

How do steroids work?

Steroids are either naturally or artificially created hormones. They can have significant effects on the body's growth and development if they are combined with a rigorous exercise program and proper diet. There are many different types of steroids, but the most widely used is a synthetic testosterone (the male growth hormone).

People take steroids to get the extra hormones into their body, hoping to promote faster growth and development and bulk-up the body's muscles by stimulating them to grow. Some people start taking them to either improve how they look or to improve their performance in sports. While steroids may enhance muscle mass, strength and stamina, they don't improve a person's skill or performance in sports.

Steroids come in different forms: injections, gels, oral drops, creams and pills. Be clear, however, that steroids are drugs and are only legal with a prescription. Many steroids have serious side effects such as mood swings (anger and aggression), hallucinations, high blood pressure, and stunted final adult height. Using steroids can also lead to testicular shrinkage and an inability to get an erection (impotence) in guys, increased facial hair growth and menstrual changes in gals, and even death. These days, because of both the risks and the unfair advantage that steroid users have over other athletes, most professional sports organizations ban the use of steroids.

52

What does "sexual orientation" mean?

Sexual orientation refers to what gender a person is physically, emotionally, romantically and sexually attracted to. Heterosexuals are attracted to the opposite gender, homosexuals are attracted to the same gender, and bisexuals are attracted to both genders.

Whether a person chooses his sexual orientation, or if it predetermined at birth, is not completely agreed upon. According to the American Academy of Pediatrics, "Sexual orientation probably is not determined by any one factor but by a combination of genetic, hormonal and environmental influences."[1]

[1]"Sexual Orientation and Adolescents", American Academy of Pediatrics Clinical Report. Retrieved 2007.

53

One of my testicles hangs lower than the other...is this normal?

Not to worry....this is very normal. The body is not symmetrical, and the testicles are no different. Most guys have one testicle that hangs lower than the other; it is also normal if one is slightly larger than the other. If, however, one testicle is significantly larger or harder than the other, you notice a lump, there is a change in appearance, or there is swelling or pain, see a doctor and have it checked out.

54

What is this discharge?

Let's talk about guys first. If there is discharge from the penis other than urine or semen, it is often the sign of a sexually transmitted disease. The discharge may be a little or a lot and be anywhere from clear to yellow to pale green. It may be accompanied by a rash, a need to urinate abnormally frequently, or a burning feeling when urinating. If a guy has any of these symptoms, he should see a doctor immediately for diagnosis and treatment.

Now let's talk about gals. Some amount of discharge from the vagina is normal. Every day, a small amount of fluid flows out of the vagina, carrying out old cells and keeping the vagina clean. This normal discharge may be clear or milky white and doesn't smell bad. At times, the normal discharge may get a little thicker (like during ovulation or when a gal is sexually aroused). If, however, the amount of discharge increases significantly, changes in color or smells particularly bad, it could be the result of an infection. Other symptoms may include itching, burning or irritation. If a gal has any of these symptoms, she should see a doctor for diagnosis and treatment.

If a person with an infection has unprotected sex, it is likely that the infection will get passed to the partner. So always get treatment immediately and keep yourself, and your partner (if you have one), safe.

55

How can I get past my shyness?

For guys and gals who are shy, an everyday social situation can sometimes seem insurmountable. The first thing to do to help overcome your shyness is to relax as much as you can. Next, visualize the situation (whether it is a conversation, a school function or a party) going well; visualize how you would like it to be. If you are going to be in a new place, you could even go visit the location to become more familiar with it. Next, think of topics to talk about ahead of time (have a plan to fall back on!). Finally, when you are socializing with others, remember that they are not overly focused on you, or watching you, or judging you. Relax and enjoy yourself. Slowly but surely, with more and more positive interactions, your shyness will probably start to become a thing of the past.

56

Do I have to swallow?

Any time a question about sex starts with, "Do I have to...," the answer is NO! You never have to do anything you don't want to do.

When a guy or gal talks about "swallowing", it refers to swallowing a guy's ejaculation after performing oral sex on him. The options are to swallow it, spit it out, or avoid letting it in your mouth in the first place. What you do is up to you.

A gal cannot get pregnant from performing oral sex, whether or not she swallows. STDs, however, can be transferred to and from either partner during oral sex. To decrease the risk of transferring STDs or infections, use a condom or a female condom with your partner. Safer sex is better sex!

57

What is the Morning After Pill?

Emergency contraception, otherwise known as the Morning After Pill, can help a gal avoid getting pregnant if it is taken within 72 hours of having sex (it works best within 24 hours, however). This pill is about 90% effective in preventing a gal from becoming pregnant. You can get the Morning After Pill from your doctor or at most pharmacies.

Emergency contraception is meant to be used only very occasionally, as the name implies. These pills contain the same hormones that birth control pills contain, but in higher levels.   The higher doses of hormones prevent pregnancy by (1) preventing the ovaries from releasing an egg, (2) preventing the fertilization of the egg, or (3) preventing implantation by altering the lining of the womb so a fertilized egg can't embed itself there.

The Morning After Pill is approved by the Federal Drug Administration and is safe to take.   Gals report that the main side effects are nausea and possible vomiting.

58

How do you kiss?

For someone who has never kissed or been kissed, it can look a little intimidating. How do you know when to lean in, which side do you tilt your head to, how hard or soft should it be, tongue or no tongue....it's a lot to think about! The good news is that it's much simpler than it looks.

All people kiss differently, but there are a few things you can do to help the first time go smoothly. First, relax and take a deep breath; when the time is right for you and your partner, you'll sense it.   Read your partner's body language and follow her lead. Your partner may indicate her readiness by leaning in closer, looking at you in a certain way, or putting an arm around you.   When you are about to kiss, tilt your head to one side to avoid bumping noses, and gently press your lips to hers.

That's all there is to it.   After a few times, it will feel natural and you'll wonder why you ever worried in the first place!

59

What is anal sex?

Anal sex is when a guy inserts his penis into his partner's anus. The anus has thousands of nerve endings in and around it that make it very sensitive. Some people enjoy being stimulated in this erogenous zone and other people don't; both viewpoints are common.

Guys and gals who engage in anal sex will find it more comfortable if they use lubrication. Otherwise, it could hurt because the anus doesn't produce enough lubrication on its own to make sex comfortable. Be sure to use a water-based lubricant that won't break-down the condom.

60

I'm unclear about my sexual orientation...what do I do?

If you're not sure about your sexual orientation, give yourself some more time to figure it out. With time, you will begin to notice yourself becoming attracted to people and your orientation will "show itself". There is no right or wrong orientation; it is what is right for you. Some guys and gals are very sure about their orientation early on, while for others it takes time, doubt and exploration. Discover your feelings and you'll soon discover your orientation. No matter what your orientation is, remember that it is the right orientation for you and it's great that you discovered it.   Being comfortable and happy with yourself (self acceptance) is very important.

61

What's the best way to prevent catching an STD?

The best way to prevent getting a sexually transmitted disease is to practice abstinence (not having vaginal, oral or anal sex). For guys and gals who are sexually active, there are ways to minimize the risk of catching an STD:

- Choose a partner who has limited her number of previous partners and keep your number of partners limited, as well.

- Ask your partner if she is currently uninfected and only having sex with you. Keep in mind that she could have an STD and not yet know it; sometimes symptoms of an STD don't appear right away.

- Talk with your partner about safe sex, her sexual history, and care she has taken (or not) in the past to prevent infection. If you can't talk openly about these things to prevent the possible spread of an STD, rethink if you are ready to have sex with this person.

- Use a condom. This is very important and will significantly reduce the risk of transferring an STD. However, be aware that a condom may not cover the entire infected area of a person. So, while a condom is great protection, it is not foolproof. That is why talking to your partner and choosing a safe partner are such important considerations.

- Do not use a spermicide; they are no longer recommended. Spermicides can actually irritate the tissue in the vagina and make it easier to transfer an STD.

- Get regular (at least yearly) exams to ensure you are uninfected. If you are infected, you must tell your partner immediately so she can get medical treatment as soon as possible.

It should be noted that some STDs are transferred through actions as simple as kissing (herpes, for instance) or heavy touching (genital warts can be transferred this way). While it is unrealistic to think that guys and gals will abstain from kissing and touching for the rest of their lives, if you choose a partner carefully and know her history, you will continue to reduce your risk of catching an STD. If you think you've been exposed to an STD, see your doctor immediately.

62

What makes a penis get erect?

An erection is sometimes called "a boner", even though there is no bone in the penis. The penis is made of soft, spongy tissue which contains lots of small blood vessels and nerve endings.

When a guy is sexually aroused, the blood vessels in the penis fill with blood. This causes the penis to swell and grow in size. It also causes the previously soft penis to become hard and rise up. This is what is known as an erection. Once a guy ejaculates, or if he becomes un-aroused, the penis will go back to its normal flaccid, or limp, state.

63

What's a clitoris and is it important?

The clitoris is a female sexual organ. Its sole purpose is to bring about sexual pleasure and orgasm in gals. It is considered, in some ways, the female equivalent of a guy's penis. The clitoris has approximately 8000 nerve fibers (about twice as much as the penis), and therefore stimulating it can feel exceptionally good to some gals. Other gals find it almost too sensitive and prefer that the clitoris not be directly stimulated.

The clitoris is protected by a clitoral hood, which is a fold of skin that covers it. This hood is located just below the folds of the labia minora, at the very top where they come together. While the size of the clitoris varies from gal to gal, it is approximately the size of a pencil eraser and protrudes slightly when aroused. When orgasm takes place, muscles around the clitoris and vagina contract rhythmically. So, yes, the clitoris is important!

64

Do gals ejaculate?

This is a topic of controversy; some people say yes and some say no. When a guy experiences the feeling of an orgasm, he ejaculates (or ejects semen). When a gal has an orgasm, she does not usually eject fluid. Her body will produce lubrication as she is stimulated and aroused during sexual activity, but this is different than ejaculating. Some research suggests that gals can and do ejaculate, but only a small percentage of gals say that they have. Very little medical research has addressed where the ejaculate (if there is any) originates from, but gals who report ejaculating say that it comes out of the urethra. Regardless of whether or not gals ejaculate, they definitely experience orgasms and all of the pleasurable feelings associated with them.

65

How often do people have sex?

This answer will vary greatly from person to person. On average, guys and gals who are in a committed relationship report having sex about two to three times per week. That said, some people haven't had sex in years while others have sex multiple times per day. There is no "normal" in this area; it is whatever is you and your partner decide upon.

66

If I talk to my doctor about having sex, will she tell my parents?

Every state has different guidelines that doctors must follow when it comes to keeping conversations they have with teen patients confidential. For example, one state may require the patient to be older than twelve for conversations to be confidential, while another state may require the patient to be fifteen. The best way to definitively know if your doctor will keep your conversations confidential is to call the doctor's office and ask her. Also be sure to ask under what circumstances she might have to share (by law) information you tell her. The doctors or office staff will be happy to tell you about their policies.

67

Does the withdrawal method work?

Also called "pulling out", the withdrawal method is when a guy removes his penis from the vagina just before he is about to ejaculate. It is a very unreliable form of birth control. First, pre-ejaculate could still get the gal pregnant. Second, hoping the guy pulls out in time is risky. Third, even if the guy ejaculates outside the vagina, anytime there is ejaculate near the vulva, there is a risk. Finally, this method doesn't provide any protection against STDs. So although pulling out can work, it is very unreliable and unsafe.

68

How do I tell my mom that I'm ready to have sex?

Good for you for wanting to talk about such an important decision. That you are ready to discuss your choice with a trusted adult goes to show that you're thinking maturely.

Be straightforward about your thoughts, feelings and actions. Hit on the big points: that you want to be honest with her and keep her in the loop about your life, that you are smart enough to use protection every time you have sex, and that you have thought about the different possible consequences of your actions, like pregnancy and STDs. (If you haven't thought of these things, you're not ready to have sex, yet!) Be prepared for her to ask you questions about what you've said and also be prepared to give her some time to think about your answers. After all, while you've probably been thinking about this conversation for a while, it may come as a surprise to her!

69

What is a French kiss?

A French kiss is when partners touch their tongues to each other's lips, tongue and inside of the mouth. It is a very passionate kiss and often lasts longer than brief kisses on the lips.

Generally, STDs are not spread by kissing, but because more saliva is exchanged during a French kiss, the chances of catching an STD are higher than they are with a less intimate kiss. Herpes and mononucleosis (mono) are two examples of orally transmitted diseases that can be spread through French kissing.

70

How can I ask my partner to get tested for STDs?

Talking about getting tested for STDs can be uncomfortable at first, but if you can't talk to your partner about it, you aren't ready to have sex. So, be upfront with your partner. Tell him that you want to keep both you and him safe. Tell him that you want to talk about infections that, if transferred, could stay with you for your entire life. Also tell him that risking your health is unnecessary and that getting tested is a sign of maturity, respect and preparedness to engage in sex.

Finally, remind your partner that many new infections don't show symptoms right away and that old infections sometimes don't reappear for a long time, even though they are still there. If your partner doesn't want to get tested, don't have sex with him; you'd only be putting yourself at risk.

71

Does masturbating have any long-term, negative effects?

Masturbation is a safe, common and healthy sexual act. It is also nothing to feel guilty about. Most people, both guys and gals, masturbate; some may try it just once, others may masturbate every day. For "99%" of the population, masturbation has no negative side effects and is perfectly healthy (just like with any behavior, however, if it begins to interfere with your normal, daily activities, it is not good for you).

The myths that masturbating can lead to blindness, hairy palms or even death, are all completely false. In fact, some reports even suggest that masturbation has health benefits such as temporary relief of stress, depression and insomnia (the inability to sleep).

72

Does the size of a guy's foot really predict his penis size?

No, not at all. This is a common myth, but it is not true in any way. You also can't predict penis size from the size of a guy's nose or hand, or his height, weight or build.

73

Are my labia normal?

Labia are the lip-shaped folds of tissue on either side of the vulva (the female external genitalia). There is an outer pair of labia (labia majora) and within them, on either side of the vaginal opening, is an inner pair of labia (labia minora). Many gals wonder if their labia are normal, or not, because labia can look very different from one gal to the next.

The outer labia are covered with pubic hair and are soft, fatty and can be somewhat plump, while the inner lips are generally thinner. Beyond that, there is a wide range of differences in how labia appear, and all are "normal". Labia differ in:

- Size – plump or thin, long or short
- Texture – smooth or bumpy, loose or elastic
- Color – darker, pinker, or the same color as the surrounding skin
- Shape – flat or ruffled, closed or lying farther apart

Also, some inner labia protrude through the outer labia while others don't. Sometimes, too, the labia are asymmetrical and a person has a large lip on one side and almost none on the other. All of these variations in the appearance of the labia are common and normal.

74

Does drinking a beer get you less drunk than drinking a shot of liquor?

This question is a little complicated.

A standard serving of beer is 12 ounces (can, bottle, or poured), of wine is 5 ounces, and of liquor is 1½ ounces (in a mixed drink or a straight shot). Assuming that the liquor is 80 proof (40% alcohol), then each of the drinks contain the same amount of alcohol. So, you say, if they contain the same amount of alcohol, then "a drink is a drink is a drink" and they would each get you drunk at the same rate, right? In theory this is right, but in reality and every day practice, it is wrong.

Even though the drinks contain the same amount of alcohol, the truth is that they are not all the same. One reason is that that beer fills you up faster because you are drinking more liquid to get the same amount of alcohol; therefore, your body will be full on beer before it will on wine or liquor. Another difference is that you can drink a straight shot of alcohol faster than a beer or a glass of wine. People drinking shots may therefore feel the effects sooner. Also, a beer either comes in a 12 ounce bottle or is poured into a 12 ounce glass, ensuring that each one is 12 ounces. With liquor, if a bartender doesn't measure how much is being poured, a lot more than 1½ ounces can get poured into a mixed drink. Finally, not all alcohol is 80 proof; a lot of alcohol is actually stronger and is therefore more potent.

No matter what you drink, remember that the legal drinking age in every state is 21. And never, ever drive if you've had a drink. If you do, you are risking both your life and others'.

75

What is an aphrodisiac?

An aphrodisiac is anything that arouses or increases a person's sexual desire. It could be a food, drink, scent, attitude, or even the moon's cycle. While there isn't any medical evidence to support the claim that over-the-counter items (as opposed to prescription medications) can increase sexual desire, a lot of people feel they do. Oysters, licorice, power, perfume, rhinoceros horn, chocolate, a full moon, and figs are examples of what some people consider natural aphrodisiacs.

76

People make fun of me a lot...what can I do?

Unfortunately, many guys and gals are teased these days. The pain and embarrassment that comes with teasing can do a lot of damage to a person's self esteem and happiness. There are two ways to decrease the harmful effects of teasing: (1) decrease the teasing itself, or (2) decrease the effect it has on you.

It would be great if you could simply go to the teaser and say, "Hey, that hurts my feelings, please stop." It is an honest, direct and mature approach and, hopefully, would stop the teasing. However, in case that approach doesn't work, let's discuss some other options. First, try disarming teasers by taking away their "ammunition"; when they tease you, ignore them. It won't be easy, but if you don't react to their meanness, they will probably get bored and soon stop the teasing. You could also try responding with humor and make a joke of the situation.

If these alternatives don't decrease their teasing, ask an adult for help. Pick an adult who will listen to your concerns and feelings – one who will address them. If you don't get the help you need, go to another adult and *ask again*. Teasing is a big issue and sometimes the first person you tell may not understand how much pain it really causes you. Ask for an adult's help until one successfully helps you stop the teasing.

In addition to decreasing the teasing itself, you can also work on decreasing the effect it has on you. First, realize that anybody who is being mean is most likely in a lot of pain themselves (maybe they are teased at home or at school or maybe they're insecure).

People who are happy do not try to make others unhappy; only people who are hurting try to hurt others. So realize that the teaser is a sad person who is hurting. Next, be confident about who *you* are. Tell yourself how great you are and *know* that you are great, no matter what a teaser may say about you. There will always be sad people who try to make others sad; you can't lead your life allowing their words to determine your happiness level and how you feel about yourself. If you do, your happiness will always depend on somebody else's mean mood! And if you listen to the teasers who only have negative words for people, you will miss out on knowing all the positive and wonderful things about yourself. Know who you are and don't let them take that from you. Finally, stay in control of your behaviors and feelings and focus on more positive things. Remember, try to both lessen the teasing and lessen the effect it has on you!

77

What is the difference between HIV and AIDS?

HIV stands for Human Immunodeficiency Virus. It is the virus that causes AIDS. HIV is transferred when blood, vaginal fluids, semen or breast milk of an infected person contacts an uninfected person's mucous membranes or an area of broken skin (a cut, for example). Areas that are made of mucous membranes include the vagina, the opening of the penis, anus, mouth, nose and eyes. HIV can also be transferred from a mom to her baby during pregnancy, childbirth, or breastfeeding. Some other examples of ways HIV can be transferred are: sharing drug needles, unprotected vaginal, anal or oral sex with an infected partner and getting infected blood in a cut.

AIDS stands for Acquired Immunodeficiency Syndrome.   It develops from the HIV infection and weakens a person's immune system (the body's system that fights off infections, foreign substances and diseases). A person with AIDS will have a lot of difficulty recovering from common ailments (such as the flu) that would not normally be a problem for a person with a healthy immune system. They may also develop certain new infections or cancers.   While there are medications available that slow down the progression of the disease, there is still no cure for AIDS and people die of it every day.

*Don't hesitate to be friends with guys and gals who have HIV and AIDS. It is safe as long as no blood or body fluids are transferred.

78

I've thought seriously about suicide...what should I do?

You're already taking the first and most important step – you're realizing that you need help and support. Now, seek out a trusted adult (parent, doctor, or counselor) and tell him how you feel. Ask him to help you get the counseling and resources you'll need to overcome the sadness and despair that accompanies thoughts of suicide.

Suicide is not an answer; it is an end before an answer can be found. Wanting to die means you want a change, but make it a positive change, not a negative one. With help, you will be able to overcome the pain you are currently in and live a happier life.

If you want help but are not yet ready to talk with someone face to face, a good resource is the National Suicide Prevention Hotline. The number is 800.273.8255.

79

How much can I drink before I shouldn't drive?

You should never mix drinking and driving - ever. You may not know how lucky you are right now, with no history of ever having done it. Too many people have been in the fortunate place you are now, only to later drink and drive and regret it forever. And if you drink and drive and live to regret it, consider yourself lucky; many others have done it only once, and died. Even worse, they've drunk and driven and injured or killed someone else. After all, it's not just yourself you should consider if you drink and get in a car. You would be risking the lives of every driver and walker you pass; risking the physical, emotional and financial lives of countless family and friends – yours and the innocent victim's. Imagine killing someone and living with that guilt for the rest of your life. All of a sudden a taxi fare, or a call to you parents to come get you, doesn't seem so bad.

In most states, if you've had even one drink, you are probably over the legal alcohol limit and it would be illegal to drive. Your exact tolerance would depend on factors such as weight, how many drinks you had, and how long it had been since your last drink. It is safe to assume, however, that one drink will put you in jeopardy.

The ironic part is, alcohol often makes many people feel invincible, even as it is impairing their senses! So make an agreement with yourself, when you're sober, to never drink and drive. Will it be hard to call your parents, tell them you've been drinking, and ask for a ride? Of course, it will. Will you be in trouble? Maybe, but even if they are upset that you drank, they will probably be proud of you for making a good decision not to drive.

*It goes without saying that if you've used drugs, the same advice applies.   Also, remember to never be the passenger in a car with a driver who has been drinking or using drugs.

80

Which helps cure a hangover faster – aspirin or coffee?

Neither, really. Hangovers are the disagreeable physical effects of drinking too much alcohol in too short a time. They only get better with time, rest and liquids. Time is needed for your body to metabolize the alcohol and to get rid of it; rest is needed so your body can recuperate from the beating it went through; liquids (water, Gatorade or juices) are needed to rehydrate your dehydrated body. Symptoms of a hangover include: headaches, sensitivity to light and sound, weakness, dehydration, red eyes, nausea and vomiting, irritability, dizziness, thirst, body aches and diarrhea.

Aspirin will help calm your headache, but that is all it will do; the hangover and all its other symptoms will still be there. Aspirin may also irritate your already upset stomach. As for coffee, it will only make you more awake; it will not make you more clear-minded or coordinated. Since rest is one of the things a person with a hangover needs most, coffee to help get rid of a hangover is not a good idea. Remember - time, rest and liquids.

81

What does "popping the cherry" mean?

"Popping the cherry" is a slang term meaning to have sex with a virgin gal. It refers to breaking ("popping") the hymen ("cherry") of a virgin.

82

How do I do a Breast Self-Exam?

Great question.　Breast Self-Exams help detect unhealthy lumps in the breasts.　While breasts are somewhat lumpy to begin with, newly formed lumps or growths need to be examined and addressed.　Most lumps end up being of little or no concern, but sometimes they are cancerous.　Although breast cancer is the most common cancer women face, with early detection, many types of breast cancers are treatable.

To complete a Breast Self-Exam do the following:

- Give yourself the exam at the end of your period. Your breasts are the least tender at this time and it will be a good way to remember to do the exam once a month.

- Know what you are looking for, which is any area that looks or feels different from the rest of your breast, or any area that has changed since your last exam. Specifically, be on the look-out for an area of thickening or a firm lump.

- Begin the exam by first looking at the size, shape, texture and color of your breasts. Look first with your arms at your sides and then with them raised above your head. (It is very normal for one breast be slightly larger than the other.) Next, look for any dimpling (a small indention in the breast caused by a growing tumor that is tugging down on the skin). To do this, put your hands on your hips and press down firmly as you hunch your shoulders far forward, bend over/forward at the waist, and look in a mirror for dimples.

For the remaining part of the exam, fully examine one breast before examining the other one.

- Continue the exam by feeling your breasts. Lie on a bed with a pillow under one shoulder and extend your arm flat on the bed, at a 90 degree angle away from your body. Your hand should be up toward your head, with your arm forming an "L" to your body. Place three fingers beside the nipple, lightly push down, and make a dime-sized, circular motion. Repeat this motion, in the same spot, two more times, pushing a little harder and going a little deeper each time. Without taking your fingers off the breast, slide your fingers down a little and repeat the circular motions in the new area. Remember to circle three times in each area (lightly, deep, deeper) to examine the entire thickness of the breast. When you're done with an area, slide your fingers to the next area, going in up-and-down strips (not around the nipple), until the entire breast has been examined. You should examine from the collarbone to the bra line and from the center of the chest to the armpit. After you've examined the entire breast, lower your arm (resting it beside your body) and examine the armpit itself, feeling for any lumps. When you're done, complete the same exam on the other breast and armpit.

If you feel, or even think you feel, an abnormal area, be examined by your doctor.

*The "Susan G. Komen for the Cure" website has a fabulous video that demonstrates a Breast Self-Exam (much of this information is based on it). The site is http://cms.komen.org/bse/ .

83

How can I prevent premature ejaculation?

Premature ejaculation is when a guy regularly ejaculates sooner that he or his partner wants him to.   It affects approximately one out of every three guys.

The first thing to do to prevent premature ejaculation is to openly communicate with your partner. Talk about your expectations, desires, and how long it takes both of you to become sexually excited enough to orgasm. Also talk about what, if any, different techniques you and your partner could use to bring you both to orgasm at the same time. You could also try masturbating and ejaculating a few hours before engaging in sex so that you're not as sexually charged during sex, thereby helping delay your orgasm. If none of this helps prevent the premature ejaculation, talk with your doctor about treatments. Possible treatments may include medications, sexual counseling and learning techniques that help to delay ejaculation.

84

Can a guy, who hasn't gone through puberty, ejaculate?

A guy (or gal) who hasn't started puberty is called "pre-pubescent". A pre-pubescent guy can orgasm, but he can't ejaculate. It is only after a boy has started puberty and is producing semen that he can ejaculate. Until this time, his orgasms are referred to as "dry" because there is no discharge.

85

What is cunnilingus?

Cunnilingus is the formal term for performing oral sex on a gal.

86

Are a dildo and a vibrator the same things?

Dildos and vibrators are both sex toys that are used for sexual stimulation. People sometimes use them with a partner, or on themselves to help with masturbation.

A dildo is an object that is long, narrow and able to be inserted into the vagina (or anus); it is an artificial penis. It can look just like a penis or it can be more generic and plain in appearance. A dildo may or may not vibrate.

Vibrators can be shaped like a penis or can be one of many other shapes. They are mostly used externally to stimulate the clitoris, though some can be inserted into the vagina. A vibrator, obviously, vibrates. Since there are many vibrators that are shaped like dildos and many dildos that vibrate, people often use the names "dildo" and "vibrator" interchangeably.

87

My breasts are lumpy...is this normal?

Breasts are somewhat lumpy by nature because they are comprised of fibrous and fatty tissue, milk glands and milk ducts. These contribute to breasts being uneven in texture below the skin, which is perfectly normal. If, however, there is a distinct or protruding lump of any size, or any change to how your breasts normally look and feel, then you may want to contact your doctor. While a majority of the lumps gals find are non-cancerous, any concerns can best be addressed by a doctor.

88

She can't get pregnant, so do I need to wear a condom when having anal sex?

Yes, you definitely need to wear a condom.

You are only partially correct when you say that a gal can't get pregnant by having anal sex. While she can't get pregnant directly from having anal sex, semen can seep out of the anus and near to the vaginal opening. The sperm can then "swim" into and up the vagina and impregnate the gal. So, pregnancy is a possible consequence of having unprotected anal sex.

Another important reason to wear a condom when having anal sex is to control the spread of STDs. The anus is a high-risk area for many STDs, including HIV, gonorrhea, herpes, syphilis, hepatitis B and chlamydia. It is also an area full of bacteria, so if you are going to have anal sex, be sure to use a condom every time.

89

Is it ok to go out with my friend's ex if she was the one who dumped him?

It depends on how your friend would feel about you dating her ex, and how you would feel about yourself if you did it. Even if your friend did the dumping, that doesn't mean she didn't really care about the guy. She may still care for him, could have gone through a lot of pain in the breakup, or maybe would just feel betrayed if you went out with him. Ask yourself if you would like it if your friend went out with your ex. Would it hurt to see them together? Would you still want to hang out with her? Our suggestion is to treat your friend like you'd want to be treated and find somebody else to date!

90

Why do my parents always tell me to wait before having sex?

The decision to have sex is a huge and irreversible one. Once you give your virginity to a partner, you can never regain it. Anytime a guy or gal is considering such an enormous decision, it is natural for a parent to suggest waiting. Think of it this way...if you wait, you can always do it later, but if you have sex now, there is no going back.

Your parents want you to be sure that you are making the best decision in the long run, not the best decision for you, today. And let's face it...if you're thinking about having sex, there are some pretty strong sexual urges that are influencing you. Your parents are trying to help you think not only about the immediate urges, but about the long-term consequences, as well.

They want you to take the time to consider things like:

1. The Consequences of Becoming Pregnant and the Decisions You'd Have to Face

    a. Would you keep the baby?

    b. Could you finish school?

    c. Could you get a job to pay the bills?

    d. How would you get medical treatment?

    e. Would you be happy later, no matter what choice you made, knowing that you had to make it at such a young age?

    f. Coping with the emotional, physical, social, psychological and spiritual issues that would result from an unplanned pregnancy

2. The Consequences of Getting an STD and the Decisions You'd Have to Face

   a. Having, possibly, a lifelong and incurable disease

   b. Having to tell each and every future, potential partner about your transmittable disease

   c. The possibly painful, physical symptoms of your STD reoccurring at random times throughout your life

   d. Getting and paying for your medical treatment

These consequences and decisions are often overshadowed by the sexual urges guys and gals experience when they begin thinking about having sex. Your parents want you to take some extra time to think about your decision before you make it so that you can be sure it is the best long-term decision for you.

91

How do I come out to my parents?

First, know that every person reacts differently to big news and your coming out may take your parents some time to get used to.   Next, be aware that there are some common emotional phases that families may go through, in part or in whole, when a child "comes out".   These phases are: shock, denial, guilt, expression of their feelings, making a decision, and true acceptance. Some families never experience the first three stages while others never experience the last.   Every family's ability to be supportive is unique, but knowing the general phases your family may go through will benefit everybody. Finally, be patient. It has probably taken you a while to be sure of your sexual orientation and it may take your parents a while, too.

In some circumstances it may be best to not come out to your parents, yet. If you think they may cut ties with you, that coming out would do irreparable damage to your relationship, or that extreme other consequences may occur, you may want to wait until you feel the situation is better before coming out.

If, however, you have determined that it is the right time to come out, tell your parents directly, confidently, and honestly. Tell them the truth - that you are proud of who you are and that you would like their support, love and understanding. Pick a time when you can talk without interruption or distractions and be prepared to answer a lot of questions.

Two great websites that have a lot of this information, and more resources and links to supportive organizations in your area, are www.outproud.org and www.pflag.org .

92

Where can I get free birth control?

Free condoms are available from a number of sources, but you may have to search a little to find them. Schools often offer free condoms through the school nurse. If your school doesn't, the nurse will be able to direct you to where you can get them in your area. Also, many clinics offer free condoms. You can call your state's Department of Health to get contact numbers for clinics near you. Other birth control, such as the pill, diaphragm or IUD, is available by prescription only and is not given out for free.

93

How many times can a gal orgasm during sex? A guy?

Having a second orgasm (or third, or fourth...) soon after the first one, without the body relaxing in-between, is referred to as having "multiple orgasms". It is common for gals to experience multiple orgasms because their bodies can "recover" between orgasms fairly quickly. That said, it is also just as normal for a gal to never have a multiple orgasm; it just depends on the gal.

Guys can also have more than one orgasm during sex, but they usually have just one because they require a longer time to recover between orgasms.

94

I heard pot isn't as dangerous as some other drugs...true or false?

Marijuana, or "pot", has often been suggested to be one of the "safer" drugs and there are some studies that support this theory. However, having fewer dangerous effects than cocaine and heroin does not mean marijuana is safe; it just means it is safer than other extremely harmful drugs.

Pot is illegal in every state. Smoking it can alter a person's brain, resulting in changes to mood, perception and behavior. It can also alter a person's physical and biochemical functioning. Specifically, pot can impair memory and the ability to learn, increase heart rate, decrease problem solving skills, and injure or destroy lung tissue (causing many of the same respiratory problems that cigarette smokers have). It can also distort thinking, decrease motor coordination, increase anxiety, lower a person's sex drive, delay reaction times and decrease the sperm count in guys. While pot may not technically be as risky as some other drugs, it is still a very dangerous, harmful and illegal drug.

95

How do I use a female condom?

A female condom is a sheath of polyurethane that gals wear during sex to protect against pregnancy and the transfer of STDs. They are 95% effective if used correctly and are best if used for vaginal sex only (they are difficult to use for anal sex). Female condoms are about 6.5 inches long, have a ring on either end, and are pre-lubricated to make it easier to insert into the vagina. It is safe to add more lubricant to the condom, if needed. A distinct advantage of the female condom over a male condom is that it can be inserted in advance of a sexual encounter.

To use a female condom:

1. Check the expiration date.

2. Remove the condom from its package, making sure the inner ring is inside the sheath and that the sheath is extended. If you want to add more lubricant, do so.

3. Grasp the inner ring and pinch it into an oval shape.

4. Keep the ring pinched and insert it far enough into the vagina that it doesn't pop out.

5. Next, insert one finger into the exposed end of the condom and push it into the vagina as far as it will go. The inner ring, which has now popped back to a circular shape, will hold the condom securely in the vagina during sex. The outer ring will remain outside the vagina and secure it there.

6. Hold the outer ring in place as the penis is initially inserted into the vagina so that the penis goes into the condom and not around it.

7. When you're ready to remove the condom, pull on the outer ring, making sure not to expose your genitalia to any semen.

Figure 4: Female Condom

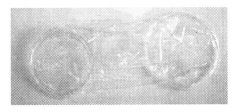

96

Does a guy have to go to a special doctor like a gal does?

In addition to their general doctor, most gals begin seeing a gynecologist at some point in their lives. A gynecologist is a doctor who specializes in health care for women. Gals go to a gynecologist for annual check-ups, to discuss any concerns they may have, and to get prescription birth control. Guys do not have an equivalent specialist; unless he has a medical concern, a guy's annual visit with his general practitioner is usually enough.

97

I said "no" to sex and my partner didn't stop. What do I do now?

Tell a trusted adult, immediately. Tell your parents, your doctor, your school nurse or counselor, a trusted neighbor, a teacher... anybody, but tell them immediately. You will need the advice and guidance of an adult that can help you get the emotional support and medical treatment you need. Some of the help you may want is time sensitive, like the Morning After Pill (taken to avoid becoming pregnant). Other support and treatment may not be as critically time sensitive, but it is still very important to get. You will need support as you cope with your emotions, possible medical issues and possible legal issues. Tell someone you trust, someone who can help you get the resources you will need to address, cope, heal and move beyond this.

98

Can a gal get pregnant if a guy ejaculates next to her in a pool?

No. A gal cannot become pregnant if a guy ejaculates near her in a pool, even if it is very near. Being close to semen is not enough to get a gal pregnant; the semen would have to come in direct contact with her vulva for there to be a chance of pregnancy.

If, however, a gal has sex in a pool, she *can* get pregnant. Having sex in a pool, shower, or jacuzzi does not prevent a gal from getting pregnant; that is a myth.

99

Can I really die from huffing?

Absolutely. In fact, approximately 100 guys and gals die from huffing every year and countless others do permanent harm to themselves.

Huffing is when a guy or gal inhales common, household chemicals in order to get high. Its use is on the rise because guys and gals underestimate the risks, it's easy to access, and parents often don't know what huffing is so they don't readily discuss its dangers.

Inhalants can be found throughout any house. Commonly abused inhalants include: gasoline, rubber cement, nail polish remover, glue, and lighting fluid. Other common inhalants are markers, aerosol from vegetable cooking sprays, spray paint, whipped cream and compressed air (like the kind used to blow dust off computers). Warning signs that a guy or gal is huffing may include: regular purchases of a common inhalant for no apparent use, paint stains on clothing, fingers or the mouth, a chemical smell on the breath, watery eyes, and a dazed or dizzy appearance.

The dangers of huffing are dramatic. When huffed, inhalants depress the central nervous system, thereby giving the user a "rush" that is quickly followed by wooziness. Users sometimes pass out completely and suffocate on the bag they were huffing from. They can also die of cardiac arrest because the inhalants cause an irregular heartbeat. If the users don't die, they may face permanent brain damage (including cell death, memory impairment and learning disabilities) or damage to their heart, liver, kidneys and other organs. They may also permanently impair their vision, speech, coordination and hearing. The risks of permanent, physical damage or sudden death are prevalent with each and every use. Whether it's the first huff or the hundredth, every time a user huffs, he is risking his life.

100

How long does sex usually last?

There is no set answer to this because there is no "usually" when referring to how long sex lasts. Some guys and gals begin with foreplay and continue for hours. Others may want to orgasm as fast as possible and be done in a matter of minutes. The same couple who had a marathon 8 hours of sex last week may have a two-minute "quickie" next week. How long sex lasts is a decision that partners make each time they have sex.

CITATIONS

Figure 1:
Body Mass Index Values for Use With Ages 2–20 Years.
Adaptedfrom
http://www.cdc.gov/nccdphp/dnpa/bmi/00binaries/bmi-tables.pdf.

Figure 2:
Body Mass Index Chart for GALS. Adapted from
http://www.cdc.gov/nchs/data/nhanes/growthcharts/set3/chart%2016.pdf.

Figure 3:
Body Mass Index for GUYS. Adapted from
http://www.cdc.gov/nchs/data/nhanes/growthcharts/set2/chart%2015.pdf

Figure 4:
Female Condom. [Online Image]. Available
http://commons.wikimedia.org/wiki/Image:Pr%C3%A9servatif_f%C3%A9minin.jpg, 2006.
Some rights reserved. See http://creativecommons.org/licenses/by-sa/2.0/fr/deed.en_GB for specific licensing information. Author: Ceridwen.

EASY GLOSSARY

Abstinence: not having vaginal, oral or anal sex

AIDS: Acquired Immune Deficiency Syndrome; a disease of the immune system that increases a person's vulnerability to infections

Anal Sex: when a man inserts his penis into his partner's anus

Anorexia: an eating disorder characterized by a fear of becoming fat, a distorted body image, an unwillingness to eat and excessive dieting; anorexia nervosa

Aphrodisiac: anything that arouses or increases a person's sexual desire

Bulimia: an eating disorder characterized by binge eating followed by self-induced vomiting that is meant to prevent weight gain

Circumcision: the act of cutting the foreskin off a newborn's penis

Clitoral Hood: fold of skin that covers and protects the clitoris

Clitoris: female sexual organ that is very sensitive and becomes stimulated by sexual touch; in relation to sensitivity and arousal, it is the female equivalent of a penis

Cold Sore: a blister on the lips or mouth that is caused by herpes simplex; fever blister

Coming Out: to publically acknowledge being homosexual

Cum: semen; ejaculate

Easy Glossary

Cunnilingus: the act of performing oral sex on a gal

Depression: a state of despair that lasts for more than two weeks and is so severe that it disrupts a person's life; extreme unhappiness

Dildo: an artificial penis

Douching: when a gal squeezes a mixture of water and either a mild soap or vinegar into her vagina to cleanse it

Ejaculation: when semen is ejected from the penis

Erection: an erect penis; a penis that has grown, become hard and risen up in response to sexual arousal

Fellatio: the act of performing oral sex on a guy

French Kiss: when partners touch their tongues to each other's lips, tongue and inside of the mouth

G-spot: a highly sensitive area in the vagina that is especially responsive to sexual stimulation

Gynecologist: a doctor who specializes in health care for women

Hangover: the disagreeable physical effects of drinking too much alcohol in too short a time

Hickey: a temporary bruise that is left on the skin from forceful sucking or biting while kissing

HIV: Human Immunodeficiency Virus; the virus that causes AIDS

Huffing: when a person inhales common, household chemicals in order to get high

Hymen: a very thin and flexible membrane or tissue that stretches across the opening of the vagina, partially covering it

Immune System: the body's system that fights off infections, foreign substances and diseases

Impotence: An inability to get an erection

Insomnia: the inability to sleep

Morning After Pill: emergency contraception that is taken soon after sexual intercourse in order to prevent pregnancy

Labia Majora: outer lips of the vulva

Labia Minora: inner lips of the vulva

Oral Sex: when a person's mouth or tongue is used to stimulate another person's genitalia

Orgasm: the euphoric, emotional and physical sensations that are felt at the end of the sexual arousal when built-up muscle tension in the body is released; the climax of sensations that have been brought about by sexual excitement; the release of built-up muscle tension in the body that is a result of sexual arousal

Ovulation: when a gal's body produces and releases an egg

Perineum: area of skin between the vaginal opening and the anus in gals, and the scrotum and anus in men

Pre-ejaculate: the clear, slippery and slightly thick fluid that comes out of a penis when a guy is sexually aroused

Pre-pubescent: a person who has not started puberty

Puberty: the physical transition of a child into an adult that is capable of reproduction

Semen: ejaculate; cum

Sexual Orientation: what gender a person is attracted to

STD: Sexually Transmitted Disease; any disease contracted through sexual intercourse or sexual contact

Steroid: naturally or artificially created hormones

Testes: plural of testicle; the part of the male genitalia that is commonly referred to as "the balls"

Vagina: the moist canal in gals that leads from the uterus to the vulva

Vibrator: a vibrating sex toy that is used for stimulation (often of the clitoris)

Virgin: a person who has never had sex

Vulva: a gal's exterior genitalia; the full exterior anatomy of a gal

Wet Dream: an erotic dream that culminates in orgasm and ejaculation in guys

INDEX

Acne, 56-57

AIDS, 168-169

Alcohol, 162-163
  and driving, 172-174
  effects, 52-53

Anal Sex, *See Sex, Anal*

Anorexia, 74-76
  help for, 84-85

Aphrodisiac, 164

Birth Control, 150
  age requirements, 86-87
  for free, 198
  types, 46-47

Body Mass Index, 22-26

Breasts, 188

Breast Self-Exam, 178-181

Bulimia, 74-76

Circumcision, 91-92

Clitoris, 143-144

Cold Sore, 58-59

Coming Out, 196-197

Condoms, 105
  and anal sex, 189-190
  and oral sex, 37-38
  age to buy, 21
  as protection, 40-41, 189-190
  female, 203-205

Condoms, con't.
  types, 93-96
  use, 79-80, 97-100

Contraception, *See* Birth Control

Cum, *See* Semen

Cunnilingus, 65, 185

Depression, 63-64

Diet Pills, 72-73

Dildo, 186-187

Discharge, 124-125

Douche, 48-49

Drugs, 201-202

Ejaculation, 33, 184, 209
  female, 145-146
  premature, 182-183

Erection, 141-142
  spontaneous, 66-67

Fellatio, 65

Friendship, 89-90, 191-192

G-spot, 101-102

Hangover, 175-176

Hickey, 118

HIV, 42-43, 168-169

Huffing, 210-212

Hymen, 82, 106-107, 177

Kissing, 132-133
  French, 153-154
  spread of disease, 42-43

Labia, 160-161

Masturbation, 157-158

Morning After Pill, 104, 130-131

Oral Sex, *See* Sex, oral

Orgasm, 15-16, 18-19, 33-34 199-200

Ovulation, 18-19, 29-30

Penis, 141-142

appearance, 91-92, 111-113

size, 39, 159

Pre-ejaculate, 54-55

Pregnancy, 48-49, 108-110, 116-117, 209

consequences of, 194

while having period, 29-30

without orgasm, 18-19

Puberty, 184

delayed, 31-32

signs of, 50-51

Semen, 62

Sex, 147, 148-149, 151-152, 213

abstinence, 46, 86, 138

anal, 134-135, 189-190

answers about, 60-61

consequences of, 193-195

first time, 17, 81-83, 106-107

oral, 37-38, 42-43, 65, 128

See also Cunnilingus

preparedness, 69-71

Sex, con't.

unprotected, 103-105

waiting, 193-195

Sexual Orientation, 121-122, 136-137

Sexually Transmitted Disease, *See* STD

Shyness, 126-127

Smoking, 68

STD, 77-78, 103-105

prevention, 37-38, 138-140

testing, 44-45, 155-156

Steroids, 119-120

Suicide, 170-171

Tampon Use, 27-28

Teasing, 165-167

Testicles, 123

Vagina, 111-113

Vibrator, 186-187

Virginity, 27-28, 88

and infections, 77-78

Voice Cracking, 35-36

Weight Loss, 114-115

Wet Dream, 20

Printed in the United States
200213BV00001B/136-1524/A

9 780615 165189